Published By Robert Corbin

@ Irving Taylor

The Benefits of a Carnivore Diet: Boost Energy,

Increase Weight Loss and Healthy Carnivore

Recipes

All Right RESERVED

ISBN 978-1-990666-96-4

I0558140

TABLE OF CONTENTS

Pan-Seared Salmon

Ingredients:

- 3 tablespoons butter

- 2 tablespoons lemon juice

- 2 tablespoons fresh rosemary, minced

- 1 teaspoon lemon zest, grated

- 4 (5-ounce) skin-on, boneless salmon fillets

- Salt and freshly ground black pepper, to taste

- 1 tablespoon butter

Directions:

1. Season the salmon fillets with salt and black pepper evenly.
2. In a non-stick wok, melt the butter over medium heat.

3. Place the salmon fillets, skin side down and cook for about 3-5 minutes, without stirring.
4. Flip the salmon fillets and cook for about 2 minutes.
5. Add the butter, lemon juice, rosemary, and lemon zest, and cook for about 2 minutes, spooning the butter sauce over the salmon fillets occasionally.
6. Serve hot.

Buttered Shrimp

Ingredients:

- 3 garlic cloves, minced

- Salt and freshly ground black pepper, to taste

- 1 tablespoon fresh lemon juice

- 3 tablespoons butter, divided

- 1 pound medium shrimp, peeled and deveined

Directions:

1. In a skillet, melt 2 tablespoons of butter in a sauté pan over medium heat and cook the shrimp, garlic, salt, and black pepper for about 3 minutes per side, stirring occasionally.

2. Stir in the remaining butter and lemon juice and immediately remove from the heat.

3. Serve hot.

Barbecued Steelhead Strout

Ingredients:

- ¼ teaspoon paprika

- ⅛ teaspoon cayenne pepper

- ¼ cup barbeque sauce

- 2 pounds steelhead trout fillets

- ¼ cup butter, melted

- 2 tablespoons lemon juice

Directions:

1. Preheat an outdoor grill for medium heat, and lightly oil the grate.
2. Arrange the trout fillets on large piece of aluminum foil.

3. Whisk together the butter, lemon juice, paprika, and cayenne pepper; brush the mixture onto the fillets.

4. Cook on the preheated grill until the fish flakes easily with a fork, about 10 minutes; brush the fillets with the barbeque sauce; cook another 2 minutes.

Parmesan Cheese Puff

Ingredients:

- 1 cup grated Parmesan cheese

- 5 cups oil for deep frying

- 2 egg whites

Directions:

1. Heat oil in a heavy pot or deep-fryer to 375 degrees F (190 degrees C).
2. In a medium glass or metal bowl, whip egg whites until they just hold a stiff peak.
3. Fold in Parmesan cheese until evenly distributed. Form level teaspoons of batter into balls.
4. Fry balls a few at a time, turning once until crisp and golden.
5. Using a slotted spoon, remove puffs from oil and place onto paper towels to drain.

Beefy Taco Pie

Ingredients:

- 1 cup Mexican blend cheese (shredded, quantity divided)

- 4 large eggs

- 2/3 cup heavy cream, preferably grass-fed

- ½ teaspoon sea salt

- 1 lb ground beef (grass-fed)

- 1 packet taco seasoning (free of MSG, starches, and additives)

- 3 green onions (thinly sliced)

- ¼ cup salsa

Directions:

1. Preheat the oven to 350ºF.

2. Prepare a round deep dish or pie dish by greasing it with butter.

3. Heat a large skillet over medium-high heat. Be sure the beef is not low in fat to yield the best cooking results.

4. When the skillet is hot, add the ground beef, breaking it into small pieces with a spatula. Stir it occasionally until it is browned.

5. Drain the beef and stir in the taco seasoning. Set it aside.

6. In a medium-sized mixing bowl, stir together the eggs and the heavy cream. Stir in the salsa, green onions, ¾ cup of the cheese, and the salt.

7. Stir the prepared taco meat into the egg mixture.

8. Pour the entire mixture into the prepared pie pan.

9. Sprinkle some of the remaining cheese on top.

10. Bake the pie in the preheated oven for 35-45 minutes or until the top is brown and the pie is completely set.

11. Allow it to cool for 5 minutes before serving. Serve it with some other taco toppings or enjoy it as it is.

Organ Meat Pie

Ingredients:

- ½ lb ground beef liver

- Beef tallow, butter, or ghee

- 3 eggs

- ½ Lb ground beef

- ½ lb ground beef heart

- Sea salt

Directions:

1. Preheat the oven to 350°F.
2. Combine all of the INGREDIENTS: in a large mixing bowl. Add sea salt to taste.
3. Distribute the mixture evenly into a lightly greased 9-inch pie plate.

4. Bake the dish for about 15-20 minutes, until the egg is set.

5. Remove it from the oven, and let it cool for 5 minutes.

6. Serve warm and/or freeze in a freezer-friendly container for up to 3 months.

Angel Food Cake

Ingredients:

- ¼ tsp cream of tartar

- ⅛ cup egg white protein powder

- Stevia to taste

- 5 egg whites

- Cinnamon to taste

Directions:

1. The oven should be set to 375°F degrees.
2. Measure the egg whites and put them in a dry bowl of a stand mixer that isn't wet.
3. Add the cream of tartar to the egg whites and whip them until they form stiff peaks.
4. Add the protein powder, stevia, and cinnamon to the mix slowly.

5. Make sure you don't add too much stevia, because the sweetness could be too much.

6. Butter or tallow can be used to grease a baking dish. Do this before baking.

7. Spoon the egg white mixture into a baking dish of your choice and shape it into a cake.

8. Bake it for 20 to 25 minutes in the oven until it's golden brown on the top. Enjoy as a snack or a sweet treat.

Beefy Taco Pie

Ingredients:

- 1 cup Mexican blend cheese (shredded, quantity divided)

- 4 large eggs

- 2/3 cup heavy cream, preferably grass-fed

- ½ teaspoon sea salt

- 1 lb ground beef (grass-fed)

- 1 packet taco seasoning (free of MSG, starches, and additives)

- 3 green onions (thinly sliced)

- ¼ cup salsa

Directions:

1. To start, turn on the oven to 350oF.

2. Butter the inside of a round deep dish or pie dish.

3. Make sure the skillet is hot enough to cook a lot of food at one time.

4. When cooking beef, make sure it isn't too fat-free.

5. Add the ground beef in a hot skillet and stir it around with a spatula to break it into small pieces.

6. Stir it a few times a day until it is brown.

7. Drain the beef and mix in the taco seasoning.

8. This is how it should be done. Set it down.

9. Stir together the eggs and the heavy cream in a small bowl.

10. Mix the salsa, green onions, 34 cup of cheese, and a little salt in a large bowl.

11. Mix the taco meat with the egg mixture until it's well mixed.

12. It's time to pour all of the mixture into the pie pan.

13. Sprinkle some of the rest of the cheese on top.

14. Bake the pie in the oven for 35 to 45 minutes, or until the top is brown and the pie is done baking.

15. Allow it to cool for about 5 minutes before you serve it.

16. Serve it with some other taco toppings, or just eat it as is and enjoy it.

Easy Beef Kidney Recipe

Ingredients:

- 1 beef kidney

- Salt to taste, optional

- Butter best cold, optional

Directions:

1. Fill a small pot with enough water to submerge the kidney.
2. Cover and bring water to a boil over medium high heat.
3. Reduce the heat, add kidney and leave the lid cracked to allow heat to escape.
4. Boil for 8 minutes, monitor the heat so water does not boil over.
5. Remove from heat. Drain water and quickly rinse kidney under cool water if desired.

6. To serve, simply cut into half, medallions or bite sized pieces. Sprinkle with optional salt to taste and eat with cold butter ad libitum.

Easy Beef Heart Recipe – Carnivore Meatballs

Ingredients:

- 8 ounces ground beef heart

- 1 teaspoon salt

- 8 ounces ground beef

Directions:

1. Mix the two ground meats in a bowl until well combined. Season with salt.

2. Scoop approximately 2 ounces and roll between the palms of your hands to form a ball shape.

3. Place in a small glass baking dish.

4. Bake in a preheated oven at 350*F (175*C) for 20 minutes.

5. Juices will run onto the baking dish once meat is cooked through. Serve meatballs warm with this "sauce" spooned over.

Carnivore Quiche

Ingredients:

For the crust:

- 3 eggs

- 1 tbsp grass-fed ghee (or butter)

- 1/4 tsp sea salt

- 1 lb raw ground pork

- 5 oz pork rinds (the equivalent of 2 EPIC bags)

For the quiche:

- 8 oz bacon

- 3/4 tsp sea salt

- 3 tbsp chives (optional)

- 6 eggs

- 1 cup heavy whipping cream

- 8 oz raw cheese

Directions:

1. At medium heat, cook the bacon.
2. Once the bacon is cooked to your liking, remove it from the pan and place it on a plate to cool.
3. In a mixing bowl, whip the eggs, heaving whipping cream, and sea salt for about 1 minute.
4. With your vegetable (or cheese) grater, shred the raw cheese.
5. Fold the shredded cheese and bacon pieces into the egg-cream mixture.
6. Prepare and bake the quiche.
7. Once the crust is done baking, remove it from the oven.
8. Pour the quiche filling into the crust. It should fill to the top.

9. Finely chop the chives (if using) and garnish the quiche with the chives.

10. Bake at 375 degrees for 30-35 minutes, or until the top crisps and is a nice golden brown color.

11. Once the quiche is done baking, remove it from the oven and allow it to cool for 10-15 minutes or so. Serve and enjoy!

12. This quiche makes for great leftovers (arguably tastier than fresh!). If storing for leftovers, place the quiche in an airtight container in the fridge for 4-5 days.

Carnivore Pizza

Ingredients:

For the Carnivore Pizza Crust:

- 1 tbsp grass-fed ghee (or butter)

- 1 tbsp Italian seasoning (optional)

- 1/4 tsp sea salt

- 1 lb ground chicken (or ground meat of your choice)

- 3 eggs

- 5 oz pork rinds

For the Carnivore Pizza:

- 1 lb ground pork

- 8-10 slices pepperoni

- 1 tbsp Italian seasoning

- sea salt (to taste)

- 1 block raw cheese

- 10 pieces bacon

Directions:

Make the Carnivore Pizza Crust.

1. Follow this recipe.
2. While the crust is baking, prepare the toppings. Start by making the bacon.
3. Chop up the bacon into thin slivers (like 1/4 inch x 1 inch).
4. At medium heat, cook the bacon.
5. Once the bacon is cooked to your liking, remove it from the pan and place it on a plate to cool.
6. Make the sausage.
7. Add the ground pork to the pan with the bacon fat and increase to medium-high heat.
8. Add the Italian seasoning (if using) and salt to taste.

24

9. Cook the ground pork in the bacon fat until browned. Your goal is a nice, deep brown char. This usually takes 10-15 minutes.

10. Once the sausage is cooked to your liking, remove it from heat and leave it to cool.

11. Once the Carnivore Pizza Crust is finished baking, add the toppings to the pizza.

12. Grate the block of raw cheese over the body of the pizza crust to form a thick layer.

13. On top of the cheese, add the cooked sausage and bacon.

14. Garnish with pepperoni.

15. Bake the pizza (with the toppings) at 350 degrees for 10-15 minutes.

16. Once the toppings have melted and set, remove the pizza from the oven.

17. Let it cool for 10-15 minutes, then serve and devour!

18. This pizza is best served fresh, although it will last in the fridge for 3-4 days in an airtight container.

Meat Muffins With Hidden Liver

Ingredients:

- 1 tablespoon beef tallow or other cooking fat

- 1 teaspoon salt

- 1 tablespoon herbs de Provence optional

- 1 pound ground beef

- ¼ pound beef liver ground (see notes)

- 4 eggs

Directions:

1. Preheat oven to 350°F (177°C).
2. Mix meat and liver in a bowl.

3. Whisk eggs, pour over meat and stir to combine.
4. Melt the tallow and pour over meat egg mixture. Mix well.
5. Season with salt and optional herbs.
6. Grease a 12-cup muffin pan or use cupcake liners.
7. Spoon mixture into each well evenly.
8. Bake for 20 minutes. Remove from oven and cool for 10 minutes before taking out of the pan.
9. They may look wet still, but it's just the melted fat.
10. Let them cool and everything will firm up. Serve warm or leftovers cold.

Slow Cooked Organ Meat Stew

Ingredients:

- 1 cup mushrooms chopped

- ¼ cup parsley chopped

- ½ teaspoon whole black peppercorn

- ½ teaspoon salt

- 8 cups bone broth or water

- 2 pounds beef heart

- 1 pound beef kidney

- 1 medium onion diced

- 2 cloves garlic minced

- 1 medium cauliflower chopped

Directions:

1. Trim off any connective tissues and large vessels from the heart; cut into 1 to ½-inch cubes.

2. Cut kidney into similar sized pieces. Leave the fat on both the heart and kidney. Add to a large stockpot.

3. Arrange the onion, garlic, cauliflower, mushrooms, and parsley over the meat.

4. Season with salt. Add peppercorn.

5. Pour in bone broth.

6. Bring to just boiling on the stove over medium heat.

7. Reduce heat and maintain a steady simmer for 2-3 hours until heart is tender.

8. Crock Pot / Slow Cooker Option

9. Trim and prepare the heart and kidney. Put it in the crockpot.

10. Add the remaining ingredients.

11. Cook on low for 4-6 hours, until heart is tender.

Livers And Hearts Of Bbq Chicken

Ingredients:

- 2 pound frozen chicken hearts, room temperature

- to taste pepper

- to taste salt

- 2 pound frozen chicken livers, room temperature

- a couple of bamboo skewers that have been soaked in water for an hour

Directions:

1. Remove extra fat from the hearts and livers, as well as cleaning them.
2. In a flexible grilling basket, lay them flat.

3. Season the meat with salt and pepper.

4. Grill on a charcoal grill until desired doneness is achieved.

Chicken In A Creamy Cheesy Sauce

Ingredients:

-   Half a gallon of heavy cream

-   10 tablespoons butter (distributed)

-   1 cup shredded mozzarella cheese

-   6 thighs of chicken

-   1 teaspoon salt and half teaspoon pepper

-   1 cup bone broth from chickens

-   Cream cheese, 4 oz

Directions:

1. Heat a large skillet over medium-high heat. Allow 2 tablespoons butter to melt in the pan.

2. Season the chicken with salt and pepper. Also apply under the skin.

3. Place the skin-side down in the skillet with the chicken.

4. Cook for 6 minutes, or until the skin is golden brown. With a slotted spoon, remove the chicken and place it on a platter.

5. Fill the skillet with broth. Scrape the bottom of the pan to get rid of any sticky browned pieces.

6. Return the chicken to the pan. Cook, covered, until chicken is fully cooked.

7. In the meanwhile, prepare the sauce as follows: In a saucepan, combine cream cheese, cream, and the remaining butter.

8. Preheat the pot on low heat.

9. Stir regularly until all of the INGREDIENTS: are fully combined. Turn the heat off.

10. Add the mozzarella cheese and mix well. Continually stir until the cheese has melted.

11. Fill dishes with chicken. Serve with a cheesy sauce on top.

Bacon Wrapped Shrimp With Sriracha Mayo

Ingredients:

- ¼ cup mayonnaise

- 1 teaspoon sriracha sauce

- Bacon Wrapped Shrimp with Sriracha Mayo

- 20 jumbo shrimp (16/20 count), peeled, deveined, tail on

- 10 slices bacon, cut in half

- Sriracha Mayo INGREDIENTS:

Directions:

1. Preheat oven to 350 degrees. Line a baking sheet with foil and place the cut strips of bacon the tray.

2. Par cook the bacon until it begins to shrink and turn slightly red, about 10 minutes. The

bacon should be flexible and not completely cooked.

3. Cool the bacon until it is easy to handle with fingertips, about 5 minutes.

4. Wrap a slice of par-cooked bacon around each shrimp, slice through a pre-soaked skewer or insert a toothpick to secure the wrap.
Continue wrapping.

5. Grill the bacon wrapped shrimp skewers over direct high heat for 3 to 5 minutes on each side or until the shrimp have plumped up and are white and pink.

6. Or cook in a 400 degree oven for about 5 minutes each side.

7. To make the sriracha mayo, mix the mayonnaise and sriracha sauce together until combined.

Smoked Roast Beef

Ingredients:

- 1 2-3 lb eye of round roast

- 1 Tablespoon Hey Grill Hey Signature Beef Seasoning

Directions:

1. Preheat your smoker to 225 degrees F with a hardwood like oak, hickory, or pecan.
2. Season the eye of round roast liberally on all sides with the beef seasoning.
3. Place the roast directly on the grill grates or in a roasting pan, and cook until the internal temperature reaches 120 degrees for rare roast beef.
4. Remove the roast from the grill and increase the temperature to High (around 450-500 degrees) or preheat a cast iron pan on your stove top to High.

5. Place the roast on the hot grill or pan and sear for 2-3 minutes per side until the roast is nice and dark all around.

6. Remove the roast from the heat and rest for 10 minutes.

7. Slice thin against the grain and serve.

8. For any leftovers, allow the roast to cool until it stops steaming, then cover and place in the refrigerator until chilled (I leave it overnight).

9. Once chilled through, slice thin and serve on sandwiches.

Chicken Curry

Ingredients:

- ½ teaspoon freshly ground black pepper

- ½ teaspoon paprika

- ¼ teaspoon cayenne pepper

- 4 tablespoons tomato paste

- 3 garlic cloves, minced

- 1 tablespoon dried minced onion

- 1½ pounds chicken tenders

- ¾ cup sour cream

- 1 tablespoon garam masala

- 1 teaspoon ground cinnamon

- 1 teaspoon ground ginger

- 1 teaspoon kosher salt

- 2 tablespoons olive oil

Directions:

1. The oven should be set to 375°F.

2. It is best to put the chicken tenders in an oven-safe dish that has a lid, like this one:

3. A medium bowl is the best place to mix the sour cream, garam masala spice mix, cinnamon with salt, black pepper, paprika, cayenne pepper, tomato paste, and olive oil.

4. It's essential to ensure that each piece of chicken is covered in sauce.

5. Cover and bake for 45 minutes until the sauce is bubbling, then let it rest for another 15 minutes.

6. Serve hot. Another 12 teaspoon of cayenne pepper can make the food even more spicy!

Chicken Noodle Soup

Ingredients:

- 4 pieces

- 2 celery stalks, trimmed

- 2 tablespoons chicken bouillon powder

- 2 teaspoons kosher salt

- 1 teaspoon freshly ground black pepper

- 3½ ounces shirataki noodles

- 7 cups chicken broth, divided

- 1 cup water

- 1 large tomato

- ½ onion

- 2 carrots, peeled and each cut into

- 2 teaspoons chopped fresh parsley Poached Chicken Breast

Directions:

1. Chicken broth and water should be mixed in a large stockpot.
2. Cover the pot and bring to a boil over high heat.
3. Add the whole tomato, onion, carrot, celery, chicken bouillon powder, salt, and pepper, and stir until they're all mixed.
4. Turn the heat down to low for two hours and let it cook.
5. Before the soup is ready, make the noodles.
6. For two minutes, put the noodles in cold water and let them stay there for a while.
7. Over high heat, bring the last 1 cup of chicken broth to a boil in a small saucepan. Pour in the noodles and parsley.
8. Add the chicken and cook for two minutes, then serve.

9. Remove the onion, celery, and tomato from the soup using a slotted spoon.

10. Add the chicken, noodles, and broth to the stockpot, stir to mix them all, and then put the pot on the stove.

11. Spoon the food into bowls and serve.

12. It's a good idea to keep any soup you make in an airtight container and keep it in the fridge for up to 3 days or freeze it for up to 3 months.

Broiled Lamb Chops

Ingredients:

- 2 tablespoons fresh lemon juice

- Salt and freshly ground black pepper, to taste

- 8 (4-ounce) lamb loin chops, trimmed

- 2 tablespoons Parmesan cheese, shredded

- 2 tablespoons garlic, minced

- 2 tablespoons fresh oregano, minced

- ½ teaspoon fresh lemon zest, grated finely

- 1 tablespoon butter, melted

Directions:

1. In a large bowl, add all the INGREDIENTS: except for lamb chops and Parmesan and mix until well combined.

2. Add the chops and coat with the garlic mixture generously.

3. Cover the bowl and refrigerate to marinate for at least 1 hour, flipping occasionally.

4. Preheat the broiler of the oven to high heat. Grease a broiler pan.

5. Arrange the chops onto the prepared broiler pan.

6. Broil for about 3-4 minutes per side.

7. Serve hot with the sprinkling of Parmesan.

Grilled Salmon

Ingredients:

- ¼ cup butter, melted

- 2 tablespoons fresh lemon juice

- 4 (4-ounce) salmon fillets

- 2 garlic cloves, minced

- 1 teaspoon dried oregano, crushed

- 1 teaspoon dried basil, crushed

- Salt and freshly ground black pepper, to taste

Directions:

1. For salmon: in a large bowl, add all INGREDIENTS: except for salmon and mix well.

2. Add the salmon and coat with marinade generously.

3. Cover and refrigerate to marinate for at least 1 hour.
4. Preheat the grill to medium-high heat. Grease the grill grate.
5. Place the salmon onto the grill and cook for about 4 minutes per side.
6. Serve hot.

Deer Jerky

Ingredients:

- 3 tablespoons teriyaki sauce

- 1 tablespoon ketchup

- 1 teaspoon hot pepper sauce, or to taste

- 1 tablespoon garlic powder

- 1 teaspoon onion powder

- 1 teaspoon black pepper

- ¾ cup Worcestershire sauce

- ¼ cup soy sauce

- 1 tablespoon liquid smoke

- 1 tablespoon fresh lemon juice

- 1 pound venison, cut into 1 x 1/4 inch strips

Directions:

1. Stir together Worcestershire sauce, soy sauce, liquid smoke, lemon juice, teriyaki sauce, ketchup, and hot pepper sauce in a bowl.

2. Season with garlic powder, onion powder, and pepper.

3. Mix in the sliced venison until completely coated.

4. Cover tightly, and marinate at least 8 hours in the refrigerator.

5. Prepare jerky in a food dehydrator according to manufacturer's Directions:, or dry on racks in the oven at 150 degrees F (65 degrees C) until the jerky has dried and will snap when bent, 10 to 12 hours.

Herb Roasted Bone Marrow

Ingredients:

- Marrow bones from grass-fed/pasture-raised beef

- Fresh rosemary

- Fresh thyme

- Unrefined salt

- Ground black pepper

Directions:

1. If you have purchased frozen bones, make sure to thaw them completely in the fridge before cooking.

2. Preheat the oven to 400°F degrees. Place the bones in a baking dish or cast iron pan.

3. Using a sharp knife, chop equal parts of fresh rosemary and thyme.

49

4. You can also use ½ tsp of chopped herbs for every 4 marrow bones.

5. Sprinkle the herbs over the marrow bones and make sure each one is covered.

6. Roast the bones for about 15 minutes, or until they are no longer pink inside.

7. Season the bones with salt and pepper and serve hot.

8. Use a small spoon to scoop out the marrow.

9. You can also keep the residue liquid in the pan in an airtight container in the fridge to add to your other meals for added flavor.

Chicken Gizzards And Broth

Ingredients:

- 2 cloves garlic (chopped finely)

- 1 tsp sea salt

- ¼ tsp ground black pepper

- 4 cups water

- 1 lb chicken gizzards (cut into quarters)

- 2 tbsp ghee

- 1 medium onion (chopped)

Directions:

1. Using the sauté setting on your pressure cooker, sauté the onions, garlic, and gizzards.

2. Cook the mixture until the onions are translucent and gizzards no longer look raw,

then add in your water. Make sure to stir it
occasionally.

3. Put the lid on the cooker and cook the dish at
high pressure for 25 minutes.

4. Allow it to naturally depressurize before
opening.

5. Garnish the dish with chives and/or chive
blossoms (optional).

Organ Meat Pie

Ingredients:

- ½ lb ground beef heart

- ½ lb ground beef liver

- Beef tallow, butter, or ghee

- 3 eggs

- ½ Lb ground beef

- Sea salt

Directions:

1. The oven should be set to 350°F. In a large bowl, mix together all of the INGREDIENTS:. Add sea salt to your taste.

2. Pour the mixture into a lightly greased 9-inch pie dish.

3. Bake the dish for about 15 to 20 minutes, until the egg is cooked and set.

4. Remove it from the oven, and let it cool for about 5 minutes before eating it.

5. Serve it hot, or put it in a freezer-safe container and put it in there for up to three months to keep it cold.

Herb Roasted Bone Marrow

Ingredients:

- Marrow bones from grass-fed/pasture-raised beef

- Fresh rosemary

- Fresh thyme

- Unrefined salt

- Ground black pepper

Directions:

1. If you bought frozen bones, let them thaw completely in the fridge before cooking them.

2. The oven should be set to 400°F degrees. In a baking dish or cast iron pan, put the bones.

3. Equal parts of fresh rosemary and thyme should be cut with a sharp knife, then put in a bowl.

4. For every 4 marrow bones, you can add 12 tsp of chopped herbs to the water.

5. Spritz some spices on the marrow bones and ensure each is covered with them.

6. Roast the bones for about 15 minutes, or until they aren't pink on the inside any more.

7. Salt and pepper the bones and serve them hot.

8. Use a small spoon to get the marrow out of the bone, then put it back in.

9. You can also keep the leftover liquid in the pan in an airtight container in the fridge to add it to your other food to make it taste better.

Homemade Bone Broth Recipe

Ingredients:

- ¼ cup raw apple cider vinegar lemon, or lime juice

- veggie and herb scraps optional, see note

- 4-6 pounds beef bones from grass-fed beef, goat, or lamb*

Directions:

1. Dry roast bones at 350*F until lightly golden brown by placing the bones in a roasting pan or glass pyrex, (no butter or oil). Roast for about 20 minutes.**

2. In a large pot, add the bones and cover completely with water.

3. Pour in vinegar or lemon/lime juice.

4. Bring to a simmer over low heat and maintain for 24 hours.

5. Do not boil. Keep an eye on the water line, make sure the bones stay covered with water. Top off as needed.

6. Add optional herbs and veggie scraps like onion, carrot, celery, rosemary, thyme, and/or oregano in the last two hours of the cooking time.

7. Remove from heat and let cool a little. If there is any film on top, skim it off.

8. Strain contents through a cheese cloth or fine mesh strainer.

9. Store in the refrigerator for up to 5 days, freeze for longer.

10. To make ENDLESS broth: Strain the bones and separate what ever meaty parts you want to eat.

11. Return the cooked bones to the pot and add an additional 1-2 pounds of fresh meaty bones.

12. Begin the process again from step 2.

13. Repeat this process over and over again all week (month?) long.

14. You'll see when the bones are done; there marrow will be gone and the porous parts will have disintegrated.

15. Keep the cycle going by tossing the old bones and replacing with fresh meaty ones until you've had enough.

Carnivore Custard Recipe

Ingredients:

- 2 cups heavy cream

- 1 tablespoon vanilla extract

- 3 whole eggs

Directions:

1. Preheat the oven to 350°F (175°C).

2. Whisk all ingredients together in a large bowl until completely smooth.

3. Divide evenly between 4 2 or 3-inch ramekins and place them in an 8×8-inch baking dish.

4. Bring 2-3 cups of water to a boil in a small saucepan.

5. Create a water bath by pouring boiling water into the baking dish.

6. Continue until the water level is an inch high.

7. Bake for 30 minutes, check, and continue for 10 more minutes if needed.

8. The top should be golden brown and firm.

9. The under part will be wiggly still.

10. Remove from the oven. Let cool and set for 10 minutes, before serving warm or refrigerating until chilled. It will firm up as it sits.

Roasted Pork Loin

Ingredients:

- 1 teaspoon paprika

- 1 teaspoon ground mustard

- 1/2 teaspoon pepper

- 3 pound pork loin roast

- 2 teaspoons salt

- 2 teaspoons garlic powder

Directions:

1. Preheat the oven to 375 degrees. Allow pork loin to be at room temperature while the oven is preheating.

2. a small bowl with dry rub seasoning next to a small whisk

3. In a small bowl, mix together salt, garlic powder, paprika, ground mustard and pepper.

4. Pat the pork loin dry with a paper towel.

5. Massage dry rub all around pork loin roast.

6. Add pork loin to a baking dish with the fat cap facing up.

7. Bake at 375 degrees until it reaches a temperature of 140 F degrees, 60 minutes.

8. Remove from the oven and allow to rest for 15 minutes before slicing.

9. Slice the roasted pork loin crossways into ¾ to 1 inch slices and serve with a drizzle of the pan drippings or make a gravy.

Dairy Free Liver Pate With Ox Liver

Ingredients:

- 1 tablespoon raw apple cider vinegar

- 1 tablespoon Rosemary

- 1 tablespoon thyme

- ½ teaspoons salt

- ¼ teaspoon ground black pepper

- 1 cup coconut oil duck fat, lard or bacon fat, divided

- 1 small onion diced

- 2 cloves garlic minced

- 1 pound ox liver or beef liver

Directions:

1. Saute the onion in 2 tablespoons of cooking fat over medium heat.

2. Cook for about 5 minutes, until transparent and soft. Stir occasionally to avoid burning.

3. Add garlic and continue cooking for another 2 minutes or so until garlic is fragrant and golden in color.

4. Slice the liver into thin strips. Push the onion and garlic over to the side of the pan and arrange the liver in a single layer.

5. Sear it for 30 seconds to 1 minute on each side.

6. Remove from heat and let cool.

7. Transfer liver, onion, and garlic sauté to the bowl of a food processor.

8. Add the vinegar, rosemary, thyme, salt, and pepper. Add 1/2 cup of fat.

9. Pulse to chop liver. Blend to combine. Add the remaining fat.

10. Continue blending until smooth.

11. Put into an airtight container and chill in the fridge for 4 hours or overnight.

Easy Beef Kidney Recipe

Ingredients:

- salt to taste, optional

- butter best cold, optional

- 1 beef kidney

Directions:

1. Fill a small pot with enough water to submerge the kidney.
2. Cover and bring water to a boil over medium high heat.
3. Reduce the heat, add kidney and leave the lid cracked to allow heat to escape.
4. Boil for 8 minutes, monitor the heat so water does not boil over.
5. Remove from heat.
6. Drain water and quickly rinse kidney under cool water if desired.

7. To serve, simply cut into half, medallions or bite sized pieces.

8. Sprinkle with optional salt to taste and eat with cold butter ad libitum.

Roast Chicken With Salt And Pepper

Ingredients:

- To taste freshly ground pepper

- To taste kosher salt

- 2-3 pounds chicken, chopped into chunks (bone-in and skin on if using chicken breasts)

Directions:

1. To prepare the chicken, blot it dry using paper towels.
2. Whole chicken may also be used. Place in a mixing bowl.
3. Season the chicken with salt and pepper. Refrigerate for 1 to 8 hours.
4. Place the chicken pieces in a single layer on a roasting pan with the skin side up.

5. Roast for 30 minutes (or 50-60 minutes if using a whole chicken) at 400 degrees F, or until cooked through.

6. The temperature in the thickest section of the meat should be 165 degrees Fahrenheit.

7. Broil for a few minutes if you want the skin to be crisp.

8. Remove the entire chicken from the oven and set aside to cool. Cut and serve.

Bacon Cream Sauce With Parmesan Crusted Chicken Thighs

Ingredients:

Chicken with a Parmesan crust:

- quarter teaspoon salt half cup freshly grated parmesan cheese

- quarter teaspoon pepper 2 -3 tablespoons butter, melted (optional)

- 4 thighs of chicken

To make the bacon cream sauce:

- 3 bacon slices

- a half-tonne of sour cream

- heavy whipping cream, quarter cup

- a half tablespoon of grated parmesan

Directions:

1. In a small basin, melt the butter.

2. On a plate, combine salt, pepper, and Parmesan cheese. Mix thoroughly.

3. Butter a thigh of chicken. Shake to remove any remaining butter. Place the skin side up on a greased baking dish and dredge with the Parmesan.

4. Carry on with the rest of the chicken thighs.

5. Preheat the oven to 400 degrees F and bake the thighs for 35 to 50 minutes, depending on their size.

6. Heat a pan over medium heat for the bacon cream sauce.

7. Cook until the bacon is crisp. Remove using a slotted spoon and place aside on a dish (leaving the bacon grease in the pan). When the bacon is cold enough to handle, crumble it.

8. Whisk the cream into the skillet until it is well combined.

9. Continue to whisk until little bubbles emerge around the pan's edges.

10. Incorporate the sour cream.

11. Split the chicken between two plates. Serve by dividing the sauce among the dishes.

Poached Chicken Breast

Ingredients:

- Crispy Chicken Skins.

- 2 (8-ounce) boneless, skinless chicken breasts

- 2 cups chicken broth

Directions:

1. It's time to make some soup. In a medium-sized saucepan, mix the chicken with the chicken broth and bring it to a boil over high heat.

2. For 15 minutes, turn the heat down to medium.

3. It's time to take the pan off the heat, cover it, and let it rest for 15 minutes.

4. It's time to take the chicken out of the broth.

5. With two forks or your hands, shred the meat. Use water instead of chicken broth to make this C1-friendly.

Turkey Burger

Ingredients:

- ½ teaspoon garlic powder

- ½ teaspoon onion powder

- 1 tablespoon finely chopped fresh parsley

- ½ teaspoon kosher salt Pinch freshly ground black pepper

- 2 tablespoons avocado oil

- 1 pound 85/15 ground turkey

- 2 tablespoons grated

- Parmesan cheese

- 2 teaspoons Worcestershire sauce

Directions:

1. When you put all of the INGREDIENTS: into a bowl, mix them until they're all combined.

2. Then put the bowl in the fridge for at least an hour.

3. When you make two patties of the same size, about 12-inch thick, put them together.

4. It takes about two minutes for the oil to get hot.

5. Then, put the oil in a medium, nonstick pan and heat it medium-high.

6. Place the patties in the pan and cook them for 5 minutes, or until they are done.

7. Carefully flip the patties over and cook until they reach 165°F inside, 4 or 5 more minutes.

8. TIP: Do not flatten the burgers with your spatula as they cook, because this will let out the juices you want to keep in the burgers.

Scallops In Butter Sauce

Ingredients:

- ¼ cup chicken broth

- 1 cup heavy cream

- 1 tablespoon fresh lemon juice

- 2 tablespoons fresh parsley, chopped

- 1¼ pounds fresh scallops, side muscles removed

- Salt and freshly ground black pepper, to taste

- 4 tablespoons butter, divided

- 5 garlic cloves, chopped

Directions:

1. Sprinkle the scallops evenly with salt and black pepper.

2. In a large pan, melt 2 tablespoons of butter over medium-high heat and cook the scallops for about 2-3 minutes per side.

3. Flip the scallops and cook for about 2 more minutes.

4. With a slotted spoon, transfer the scallops onto a plate.

5. Now, melt the remaining butter in the same pan over medium heat and sauté the garlic for about 1 minute.

6. Pour the broth and bring to a gentle boil.

7. Cook for about 2 minutes.

8. Stir in the cream and cook for about 1-2 minutes or until slightly thickened.

9. Stir in the cooked scallops and lemon juice and remove from heat.

10. Garnish with fresh parsley and serve hot.

Roasted Cornish Hen

Ingredients:

- 4 (1½-pound) Cornish game hens, rinsed and dried completely

- 2 tablespoons butter, melted

- 1 tablespoon dried basil, crushed

- 2 tablespoons lemon pepper

- 1 tablespoon poultry seasoning

- Salt, to taste

Directions:
1. Preheat the oven to 375 degrees F.
2. Arrange lightly greased racks in 2 large roasting pans.
3. In a bowl, add the basil, lemon pepper, poultry seasoning and salt and mix well.

4. Coat each hen with melted butter and then rub with the seasoning mixture.
5. Arrange the hens into prepared roasting pans.
6. Roast for about 1 hour.
7. Remove the hens from the oven and place onto a cutting board.
8. With a piece of foil, cover each hen loosely for about 10 minutes before carving.
9. Cut into desired sized pieces and serve.

Salmon Jerky

Ingredients:

- 1 tablespoon rock salt

- 2 teaspoons ground black pepper

- 4 pounds salmon fillets

- 1 cup soy sauce

- 6 tablespoons brown sugar

Directions:

1. Mix soy sauce, brown sugar, rock salt, and black pepper together in a saucepan; bring to a boil and cook until sugar and salt are dissolved, 2 to 3 minutes. Remove saucepan from heat and cool marinade.

2. Cut salmon into strips, with or without the skin.

3. Pour marinade into a shallow bowl and lay salmon strips into the shallow bowl. Refrigerate for 45 minutes.

4. Preheat oven to 185 degrees F (85 degrees C).

5. Line a baking sheet with aluminum foil and place a wire rack on top.

6. Lay salmon strips on the wire rack, discarding extra marinade.

7. Place the sheet of salmon in the oven until dehydrated, about 8 hours.

Beef Jerky Trail Mix

Ingredients:

- ½ cup raw pumpkin seeds

- 3 ounces dried cranberries

- 3 ounces dried apricots, chopped

- 1 cup unsweetened flaked coconut

- 20 ounces roasted mixed nuts

- 2 (2.9 ounce) packages beef jerky, chopped

Directions:

1. Place coconut in a large skillet over low heat.
2. Heat until toasted to desired doneness, about 5 minutes. Turn heat off and let cool.
3. Place nuts, jerky, pumpkin seeds, cranberries, and apricots in an airtight container and shake to combine.

4. Add cooled coconut and shake again.

Carnivore Freezer Pizza

Ingredients:

- 2 cups mozzarella cheese

- 2 cups diced bacon

- 1 low-carb or keto tortilla (large)

- 2 tbsp ranch dressing (reduced sugar)

- 12 oz ground beef (not lean)

- 1 serving pepperoni (13 pieces)

Directions:
1. Preheat the oven to 400°F.
2. Place a tortilla on a greased baking sheet.
3. Add the ranch dressing and spread it evenly all over the tortilla surface.

4. Continue to add the cheese, beef, pepperoni, and diced bacon.

5. Make sure all of the INGREDIENTS: are spaced out evenly so that they cover the entire pizza surface.

6. Place the pizza in the oven and bake it for 15 minutes until the cheese is melted and the toppings are a light golden brown.

7. Serve warm or let it cool down for about an hour and place it in the freezer.

8. To reheat, take it out of the freezer and put it in the oven at 400°F for 5-10 minutes.

Yummy Meatloaf

Ingredients:

- 4 tbsp plain full-fat yoghurt

- 2 hard-boiled eggs (sliced)

- Sea salt and ground black pepper to taste

- 1 tsp crushed garlic

- 2.2 lb ground beef

- 1 onion (finely chopped)

- 2 large eggs (beaten)

Directions:

1. Preheat the oven to 350°F.
2. Mix together the chopped onion, beaten eggs, yogurt, and season with the salt, pepper, and garlic.

3. Add the ground beef into the mixture and stir again.

4. Lightly grease a bread tin with non-stick spray.

5. Do not use oil or butter, as this could cause the dish to become too oily.

6. Add the mixture and the sliced boiled eggs into the bread tin and put it into the oven.

7. Cook the meatloaf for one hour.

8. Let the loaf stand for 10 minutes before slicing so that it can set.

9. Serve hot or store it in the freezer for another day.

Cocoa Crusted Pork Tenderloin

Ingredients:

- ½ tsp chili powder

- 1 tbsp butter

- 1 lb pork tenderloin (trimmed)

- 1 tbsp cocoa powder (unsweetened)

- 1 tsp instant coffee

- ½ tsp cinnamon powder

Directions:

1. Preheat the oven to 400°F degrees.
2. Combine all of the spices in a mixing bowl. Prepare the pork tenderloin by removing the thin silver tendon that may be running down the centre of the loin.
3. Rub the tenderloin with butter.

4. Season the loin with all of the spice mixture.

5. Heat a cast iron or heavy-bottomed pan to high heat.

6. Spray with non-stick cooking spray.

7. Place the tenderloin in the pan and sear on both sides.

8. Transfer the pan to the oven and roast for 15 minutes or until the internal temperature reaches 145°F.

9. Remove the pan from the oven and place the meat on a cutting board and allow it to rest for 5 minutes before slicing.

10. Enjoy at any time or freeze for later consumption.

Feta Chicken Patties

Ingredients:

- 1 tbsp ground oregano

- ¼ tsp salt

- ¼ tsp garlic powder

- 1 lb ground chicken

- 6 oz feta (crumbled)

Directions:

1. Preheat the grill or oven. In a large bowl, mix all INGREDIENTS: together until they are well mixed.

2. When you roll the mixture into balls with your hands, ensure they are all the same size.

3. Press down on the balls with a fair amount of force to flatten them into patties that have been formed.

4. Repeat this process until you have 4 chicken patties left, then stop.

5. Grill or broil the patties until they reach 165°F inside, or cook them for about 7 to 8 minutes on each side.

6. Make sure they are cooked all the way through.

7. Enjoy them as part of a meal, snack, or while you're out and about. They can also be eaten on the go.

Hickory Turkey Burgers

Ingredients:

- 1 tsp parsley

- 1 tsp paprika

- 1 tsp cumin powder

- 4 tbsp liquid egg substitute or 2 large beaten eggs

- 1 lb ground turkey

- 1 dash salt

- 1 tsp liquid hickory flavored sauce (reduced sugar)

- 1 tsp garlic powder

Directions:

1. Get the grill or coals going to start cooking.

2. Add all INGREDIENTS: to a medium or large bowl and mix them well.

3. When you roll the mixture into balls with your hands, ensure they are all the same size.

4. Equal-sized patties won't break apart if you press down on the balls to make them flat.

5. Store them in the fridge for a few minutes, or carefully place them on the grill to make them crispy.

6. To ensure they are cooked all the way through, cook them for about 5 minutes on each side.

7. Use a spatula to move them around to ensure they don't fall apart as you grill them.

8. Serve and eat them right away, or save them for later and enjoy them later when you're ready.

Chicken Pops

Ingredients:

- ¼ tsp ground black pepper

- ½ tsp turmeric

- ½ tsp paprika

- ¼ cup parsley leaves (finely chopped)

- 2 lemons (halved)

- 4 large chicken drumsticks, with the skin removed (about 4 ounces each)

- 3 cloves garlic (minced)

- 1 shallot (minced)

- 1 tbsp low-sodium soy sauce

- 1 tsp mustard

Directions:

1. First, mix the first eight INGREDIENTS: and the juice of half of one lemon in a big bowl.

2. Set aside about 3 tablespoons of the mix. Preheat a grill outside to 400°F.

3. Place the chicken drumsticks on a cutting board and cut them up.

4. Use a sharp chef's knife to cut the non-meat end of the leg around the bone, turning the leg toward the blade.

5. Using small kitchen pliers, pull out the white tendons and throw them away.

6. "Lollipop": With one hand, you hold the boney end of a leg.

7. With your other hand, push the meat up toward the flesh end to make a "lollipop."

8. Scrape off the last of the flesh from the bone with a knife.

9. Repeat the same thing with the rest of the drumsticks.

10. You finish prepping them, but each one into the bowl with the marinade mixture.

11. To cook the drumsticks, put them on the preheated grill and the remaining lemon halves (flesh side facing down).

12. Turn over the drumsticks after 10 minutes.

13. Take the lemons off the grill and remove them.

14. It will take another 10 to 13 minutes on the grill to get the chicken to 165°F inside.

15. It is time to squeeze the lemons into the rest of the sauce.

16. When they're still warm, pour the sauce over them and enjoy.

Peppermint Keto Custard

Ingredients:

- 1.5 tablespoons water

- 1.5 teaspoons grass-fed beef gelatin

- 1 tablespoons powdered Monkfruit Sweetener optional

- 2 whole egg yolks raw

- 1/2 cup whole milk raw if possible

- 3/4 cups heavy whipping cream raw if possible

- 1/4 teaspoon peppermint spirits or peppermint extract

Directions:

1. Bring water to a simmer in a small saucepan.

2. Remove from heat, sprinkle gelatin over the surface of the water.

3. Set aside to sit for a few minutes.

4. Combine milk and peppermint spirits or extract. Add to water gelatin mixture.

5. In a medium bowl, whisk the egg yolks with optional sweetener.

6. Continue whisking and slowly add the peppermint milk. Continue until thickens, remove all clumps.

7. Refrigerate until thickened to a pudding-like consistency, about 30 minutes.

8. Meanwhile, beat the cream into stiff peaks.

9. Once mint mixture is chilled, gently fold in the whipped cream.

10. Refrigerate to set completely, about 3 hours.

Keto Cheeseburger Pie

Ingredients:

- ½ teaspoon garlic powder

- ½ teaspoon ground mustard

- ½ teaspoon salt

- ¼ teaspoon ground black pepper

- 1 cup shredded cheese

- 1.5 pounds ground beef

- 1 tablespoon beef tallow butter, or cooking fat of choice, separated

- 1 medium onion diced

- 4 whole eggs

Directions:

1. Preheat the oven to 350°F (176°C) and grease a 9-inch round pie plate or 8×8-inch baking dish.

2. Lightly brown the meat in cooking fat over medium-high heat in a heavy-bottomed skillet or cast iron.

3. Transfer to pie plate once cooked.

4. Add a little more fat to the skillet and brown the onions until translucent, about 5-7 minutes. Stir frequently.

5. While the onions cook, whisk the eggs. Add herbs, salt and pepper.

6. Pour over the beef so it sinks into the meat. Shake the dish gently if needed.

7. Arrange the onions in an even layer over the eggs and meat.

8. Top the whole pie with cheese.

9. Bake for 20 minutes, until cheese is melted and bubbly. Allow the cheeseburger pie to rest for 5 minutes before slicing.

Keto Nacho Sacue

Ingredients:

- 3 tablespoons shredded swiss cheese

- 1 ⅓ cup water, divided

- 1 tablespoon sodium citrate

- 7 oz sharp cheddar cheese, shredded

- 2.5 oz fontina cheese, shredded

Directions:

1. In a medium bowl, combine cheddar cheese, fontina cheese and swiss cheese. Toss until mixed.

2. In a medium saucepan, whisk together ⅔ cup water and sodium citrate over medium heat.

3. Stir until sodium citrate dissolves and the mixture begins to simmer. (Warning: Do not use a Calphalon pan.)

4. Gradually add one handful of the cheese blend at a time, stirring constantly.

5. Make sure the cheese is fully incorporated until adding the next handful.

6. Reduce heat to medium-low and whisk in remaining ⅔ cup water.

7. Stir until slightly thickened, about 2-3 minutes.

8. Mixture will continue to thicken as it cools.

9. For a thicker sauce, simmer longer. For a thinner sauce, add more water if needed.

Keto Salt And Vinegar Wings

Ingredients:

- Salt & Vinegar Marinade Ingredients:

- 1/4 cup apple cider vinegar

- 1/2 teaspoon salt

- 1/2 teaspoon garlic powder

- 1.5 pounds party wings

- 1 tablespoon olive oil

- 1 teaspoon salt

- 1/2 teaspoon pepper

Directions:

1. Pat wings dry with a paper towel. Getting excess moisture out of the wings before they bake is critical for crispy wings.

2. Toss wings in olive oil, salt and pepper.

3. Place on wire rack over a baking sheet. This will allow for air distribution under the chicken wings to ensure crisping at all angles. Bake at 400 degrees for 35 to 40 minutes.

4. In a small bowl, combine apple cider vinegar, salt and garlic powder.

5. Remove wings from the oven and toss in salt and vinegar marinade until coated.

6. Place vinegar coated wings back on the tray and broil on high for 1 to 2 minutes.

Easy Beef Heart Recipe

Ingredients:

- 8 ounces ground beef

- 8 ounces ground beef heart

- 1 teaspoon salt

Directions:

1. Mix the two ground meats in a bowl until well combined. Season with salt.
2. Scoop approximately 2 ounces and roll between the palms of your hands to form a ball shape.
3. Place in a small glass baking dish.
4. Bake in a preheated oven at 350*F (175*C) for 20 minutes.
5. Juices will run onto the baking dish once meat is cooked through.

6. Serve meatballs warm with this "sauce" spooned over.

Keto Chicken Liver Pate Recipe

Ingredients:

- 1 tablespoon parsley minced

- ½ teaspoon salt

- ¼ teaspoon ground black pepper

- ½ pound chicken livers

- ½ cup butter or duck fat for dairy free

- 1 medium shallot minced

- 2 cloves garlic minced

Directions:

1. Trim the chicken livers and remove any sinew. Kitchen scissors work well for this.

2. Melt a tablespoon of butter in a skillet over medium heat.

3. Add garlic and shallots. Cook for 1-2 minutes until fragrant.

4. Add chicken liver to the pan. Pan-fry the first side until golden brown, flip them over for the second side, about 5-7 minutes total.

5. Add parsley in the last minute of cooking.

6. Remove from heat and cool enough to add to a food processor.

7. Add remaining butter and season with salt. Puree until smooth.

8. Pour into ramekin dishes or a container and chill for 4 hours or overnight to set.

Classic Beef Liver Pate

Ingredients:

- 1/2 teaspoon salt

- 1/2 teaspoon ground black pepper

- 2 tablespoons heavy whipping cream optional, preferably raw

- 1/2 pound beef liver

- 6 tablespoons grass-fed butter divided

- 2 cloves garlic finely minced

- 2 teaspoons dried thyme

Directions:

1. Melt 3 tablespoons of the butter in a skillet.
2. Add finely minced garlic and cook on medium-high until translucent, 3-4 minutes.

3. Meanwhile, trim the connective tissue off of the liver and slice to thin strips.

4. Add beef liver to pan, increase to high heat.

5. Sprinkle with thyme, salt, and pepper.

6. Sear liver for 60 seconds on each side.

7. Remove liver from heat and let cool, about 5 minutes.

8. Transfer to a food processor or blender and puree until smooth.

9. While blending/pureeing, add the remaining butter and cream (if using).

10. Add more salt and pepper to taste, if desired.

11. Once the mixture is completely smooth, remove from blender and put in ramekins or a glass container and cover tightly.

12. Chill in the fridge for at least 4 hours or overnight (preferred) to harden and let flavors meld.

13. Serve with cucumber, celery, bacon or just a spoon.

Chicken Breasts That Have Been Pan-Fried.

Ingredients:

- To taste freshly ground pepper

- To taste kosher salt

- 1/4 cup parmesan cheese, grated (optional)

- 8 half-chicken breasts

- 2 tablespoons fat or butter

Directions:

1. Over medium heat, heat a stainless steel or cast-iron skillet.
2. Allow the butter or lard to melt in the pan.
3. Pound the chicken breasts with a meat mallet until they are evenly thick.
4. If desired, season with salt and pepper. Allow for 15-20 minutes of resting time.

5. Preheat an ovenproof skillet on high. In a skillet, brown the chicken.

6. Cook without stirring or covering for 2-3 minutes.

7. Cook until the fat has become golden brown. Cook for another 2-3 minutes on the other side.

8. Remove the pan from the heat and top with Parmesan cheese.

9. Serve after broiling for 2-3 minutes.

Chicken With A Bacon Cream Sauce

Ingredients:

- 1 cup heavy cream, double

- 4 tablespoons softened butter

- 16 bacon slices

- 10 thighs of chicken

- Half teaspoon salt and half teaspoon pepper

- 1 cup bone broth from chickens

Directions:

1. Place a skillet over medium heat. Cook until the bacon is crisp.
2. Drain any residual grease in the pan.
3. Chop into tiny pieces once cool enough to handle. Place aside.

4. Over medium heat, heat a large skillet. Melt the butter in the pan.

5. Season the chicken with salt and pepper. Also sprinkle under the skin.

6. Place the skin-side down in the skillet with the chicken.

7. Cook for 6 minutes, or until the skin is golden brown.

8. With a slotted spoon, remove the chicken and place it on a platter.

9. Fill the skillet with broth. Scrape the bottom of the pan to get rid of any sticky browned pieces.

10. Return the chicken to the pan. Toss in half of the bacon.

11. Cook, covered, until chicken is fully cooked. Set aside the chicken with a slotted spoon.

12. In the same pan, combine the cream and the remaining butter.

13. Stir regularly until all of the INGREDIENTS: are fully combined.

14. Return the chicken to the skillet and stir thoroughly. Allow it simmer for a few minutes. Turn the heat off.

15. Fill dishes with chicken. Serve with the leftover bacon on top.

Turkey Meatza

Ingredients:

- 1 teaspoon freshly ground black pepper, divided

- 2 tablespoons Italian Spice Blend

- 2 pounds lean ground turkey

- ¾ cup marinara sauce 1 teaspoon garlic salt

- ¼ cup grated Parmesan cheese

- ¼ cup chopped fresh basil

- 1 cup grated mozzarella cheese

- ¼ cup cream cheese, at room temperature

- ¼ cup egg whites

- ¼ cup almond flour

- ½ teaspoon xanthan gum

- 3 teaspoons kosher salt, divided

Directions:

1. The oven should be set to 350°F. Make sure the parchment paper is big enough to cover the edges of a 12-by-17-inch baking sheet about 2 inches on all sides.

2. This recipe is for a large bowl. Mix the cream cheese and egg whites in the bowl with a large spoon until they are all mixed and the cheese has softened.

3. Make sure you mix in the almond flour, xanthan gum, 2 teaspoons of salt, 12 teaspoon of pepper, and the Italian spice blend. Then stir until everything is mixed together.

4. With a large spoon, mix in the turkey.

5. Place the mixture on the baking sheet that has been lined with parchment paper. Gently

press it into the pan until it goes to the edges. Use your thumb to push a bit extra turkey mixture into the edges of the pan.

6. It will take about 20 minutes to bake, so remove the pan from the oven and carefully pour off any extra liquid built up. Wipe the base of the pan with a paper towel and let it dry.

7. Flatten the crust with your hands to ensure it fits in your pan all the way around.

8. Make sure the oven temperature is set to 400°F.

9. Slide the pizza crust and the parchment paper onto a large baking sheet by holding on to the parchment and carefully lifting it out of the pan.

10. Then slide the pizza crust onto the baking sheet.

11. Ensure the marinara sauce is spread out evenly over the base and doesn't cover all of it.

12. Leave the crust around the edges of the pizza dough uncooked.

13. A lot of pepper and basil should be sprinkled on the crust. Garlic salt should be sprinkled on the whole thing.

14. When it's done baking, sprinkle the mozzarella and the last 1 teaspoon of kosher salt.

15. For 2 more minutes, turn the oven on broil.

16. The meal is baking when the crust is browned and the cheese is melted.

17. 1 Serve the meatza in six pieces. Make sure the sauce has no more than 3 grams of carbs per 14 cup.

Smoky Turkey Cutlets

Ingredients:

- 1 tablespoon Smoky Spice Blend

- 2 tablespoons olive oil

- 2 (½-pound) turkey breast cutlets

Directions:

1. In a paper towel, pat the turkey dry and then rub the smoky spice blend evenly over the cutlets.

2. Heat the olive oil in a large pan over medium-high heat until it starts to smoke.

3. The heat should be turned down. It is time for the cutlets to be added.

4. Cover and cook for 3 minutes.

5. As soon as the cutlets are turned over, cover them with the lid and cook them for about 3 more minutes. TIP: Mix this dish with Dill Dip.

Grilled Whole Chicken

Ingredients:

- 3 tablespoons butter, melted

- 1 (4-pound) whole chicken, neck and giblets removed

- Salt and freshly ground black pepper, to taste

Directions:

1. Preheat the grill for indirect heat. Adjust the temperature to 350-400 degrees in the indirect area.

2. Grease the grill grate.

3. Coat the chicken with about 1½ tablespoons of butter and then season with salt and black pepper.

4. Arrange the chicken over the indirect heat, angling one thigh and leg to the direct heat side.

5. Close the grill with lid and cook for about 40 minutes.

6. Rotate the bird, angling the other thigh towards the heat and coat with the remaining butter.

7. Cook for about 40 minutes more.

8. Remove from the grill and place the chicken onto a cutting board for about 5-10 minutes before carving.

9. With a sharp knife, cut the chicken into desired-sized pieces and serve.

Chicken & Bacon Casserole

Ingredients:

- 4 (5-ounce) skinless, boneless chicken breasts

- ½ cup butter, melted

- 1 cup Asiago cheese, shredded

- 3-4 cooked bacon slices, crumbled

- 1 egg

- 1 tablespoon water

- ¾ cup Parmesan cheese, shredded

- ¼ teaspoon garlic powder

- Salt and freshly ground black pepper, to taste

Directions:

1. Preheat the oven to 350 degrees F. Arrange a rack into a foil-lined baking dish.

2. In a small shallow dish, add the egg and water and beat lightly.

3. In another shallow dish, add the Parmesan cheese, garlic powder, salt and black pepper and mix well.

4. Dip each chicken breast in egg mixture evenly and then coat with the cheese mixture.

5. In a deep skillet, melt the butter over medium-high heat and fry chicken breasts for about 3-4 minutes or until golden brown from both sides.

6. With a slotted spoon, remove the chicken breasts and arrange into the prepared baking dish in a single layer.

7. Bake for about 20 minutes or until chicken is cooked through.

8. Remove the baking dish from the oven and sprinkle the chicken breasts with Asiago cheese, followed by the bacon.

9. Now, set the oven to broiler.

10. Broil for about 2-3 minutes or until cheese is melted and bubbly.
11. Serve hot.

Roasted Turkey

Ingredients:

- Salt and freshly ground black pepper, to taste

- 1 Spanish onion, quartered

- 1 head garlic, halved crosswise

- 1 large bunch fresh thyme

- 1 whole lemon, halved

- ¼ pound unsalted butter, melted

- 2-3 tablespoons fresh lemon juice

- 2 teaspoon lemon zest, grated

- 1 teaspoon fresh thyme leaves, chopped

- 1 (10-pound) whole turkey, giblets removed

Directions:

1. Preheat the oven to 350 degrees F.

2. In a bowl, add the butter, lemon juice, lemon zest and thyme leaves and mix well. Set aside.

3. Season the inside of the turkey cavity with salt and black pepper generously.

4. Arrange the turkey into a large roasting pan.

5. Stuff the cavity with the onion, garlic, bunch of thyme and lemon haves.

6. Brush the outside of the turkey with the butter mixture and sprinkle with salt and black pepper.

7. With kitchen string, tie the legs together and tuck the wing tips under the body of the turkey.

8. Roast for about 2½ hours.

9. Remove from the oven and palace the turkey onto a platter.

10. With a piece of foil, cover the turkey for about 15-20 minutes before carving.

11. With a sharp knife, cut the turkey into desired sized pieces and serve.

Smoked Brisket

Ingredients:

- 3 tablespoons mustard, or as needed

- 2 tablespoons brisket , or as needed

- 5 pounds beef brisket, trimmed of fat

Directions:

1. Coat beef brisket with mustard. Cover with brisket rub.
2. Let marinate in the refrigerate, 8 hours to overnight.
3. Remove brisket from the refrigerator and bring to room temperature.
4. Preheat a smoker to 220 degrees F (104 degrees F) according to manufacturer's instructions.

5. Place beef brisket in the smoker and smoke until easily pierced with a knife and an instant-read thermometer inserted into the center reads 190 degrees F (88 degrees C), 6 1/4 to 7 1/2 hours.

6. Wrap brisket with aluminum foil and let rest for 30 minutes before slicing.

Slow Cooker Roasted Leg Of Lamb

Ingredients:

- 2 tablespoons Dijon mustard

- 3 cloves garlic, minced

- 1 tablespoon apple cider vinegar

- 1 tablespoon dried rosemary

- 1 teaspoon dried thyme

- 1 teaspoon sea salt

- 1 (3 pound) bone-in leg of lamb, or more to taste

- ½ cup red wine

- 1 lemon, juiced

- 2 tablespoons raw honey

- ½ teaspoon fresh cracked pepper

Directions:

1. Bring leg of lamb to room temperature, about 2 hours.
2. Pour wine into a slow cooker. Mix lemon juice, honey, mustard, garlic, vinegar, rosemary, thyme, sea salt, and pepper together in a bowl until a thick paste forms.
3. Massage paste into the lamb using your hands; gently place into the slow cooker.
4. Cook on Low, without removing the cover, for 5 hours.
5. An instant-read thermometer inserted near the bone should read 145 degrees F (65 degrees C).
6. Let lamb rest for 15 to 20 minutes.

Easy Roast Beef

Ingredients:

- 2 ½ lb top round beef roast

- 1 tsp cracked black pepper

Directions:

1. Preheat the oven to 400° F.

2. Remove the meat from the refrigerator and allow it to rest at room temperature for about 20 minutes.

3. Pat the meat dry with paper towels to remove any moisture.

4. Season with black pepper and then rub the pepper over the meat.

5. Place a cast-iron skillet or heavy ovenproof sauté pan over moderate heat.

6. Do not add cooking spray or any oil to the pan, as there is no grease required at moderate heat.

7. Sear the meat on all sides, then move the pan to the oven.

8. Reduce the oven temperature to 350°F and roast it until the internal temperature reaches 125°F; this will take about 50 minutes.

9. Remove the meat from the oven, cover with foil, and let it rest for 10 minutes before carving into thin slices.

10. Store for later consumption or enjoy throughout the day.

Easy Seafood Stock

Ingredients:

- 1 stalk celery (chopped)

- 6 peppercorns

- 4-½ cups cold water

- 4 oz shrimp shells (from about 15-20 shrimp)

- 1 tsp soybean oil

- ¾ cup onion (chopped)

- 1 leek, white and pale green part only (thinly sliced)

Directions:

1. Heat a stock pot or large saucepan over moderate heat.
2. Add the oil to the hot pan, then add the shrimp shells to the hot oil.

3. Sauté until the shells become bright pink or reddish in color.

4. Add the vegetables and stir to combine.

5. Reduce the heat to low and let it sweat for 3 minutes.

6. Add the seasonings and water and turn the heat up to high.

7. Bring the stock to a boil, and then lower the heat and simmer for 20-25 minutes.

8. Set it aside and let it cool slightly. Then, strain the stock through a fine-mesh strainer.

9. Add to a container of your preference and store it in the fridge or freezer.

Slow Cooker Carnivore Beef Stew

Ingredients:

- 6 cups bone broth

- 8 oz mushrooms (quartered)

- 1 large onion chopped

- 4 cloves garlic minced

- 2 tsp dried thyme

- 2 tsp salt

- 2 lb beef marrow bones

- 2 lb chuck roast cubed

- 2 tbsp beef tallow

- 1 tsp ground black pepper

Directions:

1. Start the slow cooker on a low setting and place the marrow bones in the centre.

2. Cube the roast and heat the tallow in a large skillet over high heat.

3. Arrange the meat in a single layer and sear on all sides. Once all the meat is cooked, add it to the pot.

4. Rinse and chop all of the vegetables, gather the herbs, and place everything in the pot on top of the meat.

5. Pour the broth over the INGREDIENTS: and season with salt and pepper.

6. Cover with the lid and cook on low for 6-8 hours.

7. Set it aside and let it cool down before freezing it in freezer-friendly containers.

8. Freeze it in separate containers and heat it up in the oven or microwave when you are ready to enjoy.

Beef Chuck Roast

Ingredients:

- 3 lb beef chuck (arm pot roast)

- 4 cloves garlic (peeled and halved)

- 1 tsp ground black pepper

Directions:

1. The oven should be set to 400°F. Cooking twine is used to keep the roast in place. Make 8 slits around the roast that are about 12 an inch wide. Put a half of a garlic clove in each slit.

2. Add some fresh ground pepper to it and put it on a rack in a roasting pan. Let it cook in the oven for about 20 minutes, then take it out and serve it.

3. Turn the heat to 325°F and put a meat thermometer in the roast. When the roast is

done, cook for another hour or so, until it's very soft.

4. Take care not to overcook the roast, because it can become complex and dry.

5. Roast is done. Take it out of the oven, and cover it with aluminum foil. Let it rest while covered for about 15 minutes before cutting or carving it into small pieces or squares.

6. Slice the meat against the grain and use the pan drippings as gravy when serving it. To store it in the fridge, ensure it has cooled down to the point where it is safe to put in there.

Lamb Chops For The Grill

Ingredients:

- 3 tbsp extra virgin olive oil

- 1 tbsp fresh rosemary (finely chopped)

- 3 cloves garlic (minced)

- ½ tsp sea salt

- 8 lamb chops (about ¾ inch thickness)

- Freshly ground black pepper to taste

Directions:

1. Prepare the grill or stovetop grill pan by heating it medium-high heat.

2. A small bowl is the best place to mix all the marinade INGREDIENTS:, so put them in there.

3. Ensure that this mixture is spread evenly on all sides of the lamb chops before cooking.

4. The lamb chops should be grilled on each side for 2 to 4 minutes until they are soft and juicy (135°F for medium-rare).

5. Chop the meat into small pieces and put them on a serving platter.

6. Let them rest for 6 to 10 minutes before you eat them.